ST. JOHN'S WORT

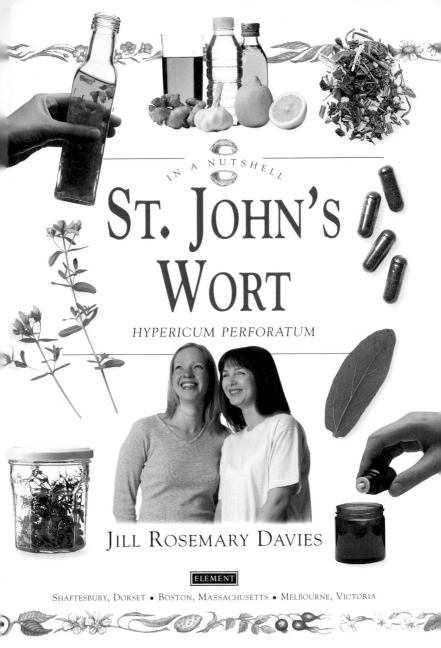

IN A NUTSHELL

ST. JOHN'S
WORT

HYPERICUM PERFORATUM

JILL ROSEMARY DAVIES

ELEMENT

SHAFTESBURY, DORSET • BOSTON, MASSACHUSETTS • MELBOURNE, VICTORIA

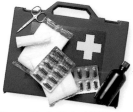

© Element Books Limited 1999

First published in Great Britain in 1999 by
ELEMENT BOOKS LIMITED
Shaftesbury, Dorset SP7 8BP

Published in the USA in 1999 by
ELEMENT BOOKS INC.
160 North Washington Street,
Boston MA 02114

Published in Australia in 1999 by
ELEMENT BOOKS LIMITED
and distributed by
Penguin Australia Ltd
487 Maroondah Highway,
Ringwood, Victoria 3134

All rights reserved. No part of this book
may be reproduced or utilized in any form
or by any means, electronic or
mechanical, without prior permission in
writing from the publisher.

NOTE FROM THE PUBLISHER
Any information given in this book is not
intended to be taken as a replacement
for medical advice. Any person with a
condition requiring medical attention
should consult a qualified practitioner
or therapist.
For growing and harvesting, calendar
information applies only to the
northern hemisphere (US zones 5-9).

Jill Rosemary Davies has asserted her right
under the Copyright, Designs, and Patents
Act, 1988, to be identified as Author of this
work.

Designed and created for Element Books with
The Bridgewater Book Company Ltd.

ELEMENT BOOKS LIMITED
Managing Editor Miranda Spicer
Senior Commissioning Editor Caro Ness
Group Production Director Clare Armstrong
Production Manager Susan Sutterby

THE BRIDGEWATER BOOK COMPANY
Editorial Director Sophie Collins
Project Editor Lorraine Turner
Art Director Kevin Knight
Designer Jane Lanaway
DTP Designer Chris Lanaway
Photography Guy Ryecart
Illustrations Michael Courtney
Picture research Lynda Marshall

Printed and bound in Great Britain by
Butler and Tanner, Frome.

Library of Congress Cataloging in
Publication data available

British Library Cataloguing in Publication
data available

ISBN 1 86204 506 2

*The publishers wish to thank the
following for the use of pictures:*
A–Z Botanical Collection: pp.6, 29, 33
  Bridgeman Art Library: pp.44, Private
  Collection. Corbis: pp.8, Tom Bean; 12t,
  Carol Cohen. Elizabeth Whiting &
  Associates: p.26c. E.T. Archive: pp.10b,
  11. Garden Picture Library: p.28. Image
  Bank: pp.28b, 45t, 55t. Science Photo
  Library: pp.12b, 19b, 27b, 47t. Stock
  Market: pp.19t, 20t. Walter Gardiner, p.13.

Contents

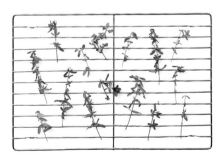

Introduction

A FAMILIAR HEDGEROW PLANT *with dainty golden-yellow flowers that appear with the longest days of summer, St. John's Wort has reemerged over the last few years as a useful herbal antidepressant.*

St. John's Wort can usually be found growing wild in woods, hedgerows, and meadows, as well as on mountainsides and roadsides. Appearing between mid-June and late August, its bright and cheery "solstice" flowers are small, numerous, and clustered together on branching pale green stems, which give an uneven, staggered, umbrella effect.

DEFINITION

Botanical family: *Guttiferae* (although botanists have recently assigned it to *Clusiaceae*).
Species: *Hypericum perforatum* is the main species used commercially for medicinal purposes and therefore, unless otherwise stated, it is the species referred to in this book. *Hypericum angustifolia* is an old favorite and is still freely harvested for home use. *H. perforatum* can be distinguished from *H. angustifolia* by its oil glands, which show up as transparent dots against the light.

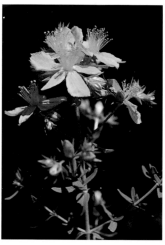

ABOVE **Hypericum perforatum – the variety used commercially.**

The herb's delicate flowers have five petals with tiny, almost imperceptible black dots along their margins. These flowers measure approximately 1in (2.5cm) across, and the cluster of stamens that protrude from their centers give them an altogether "fairy-like" effect.

THREE VARIETIES

The genus *Hypericum* contains approximately 400 different species of annuals, perennials, shrubs, and small trees, ranging from very small perennials to trees of 10ft (3m), and includes both varieties of St. John's Wort as well as *Hypericum androsaemum*, another interesting member of the Hypericum genus. A native of both sides of the Mediterranean Sea and western Asia, *Hypericum androsaemum* grows profusely in Australia and New Zealand, where it is considered to be a weed. It is commonly known as Tutsan, a corruption of *tout-sain* (meaning "all health"), which refers to the medicinal uses of the plant.

RIGHT **The leaves of St. John's Wort are pale green with tiny dots underneath.**

grown, reaching 1–3ft (0.3–1m) in uncultivated soils.

One of the unique features of *Hypericum perforatum* is its leaves which, when held to the light, show tiny translucent dots on their underside: these are the glands that contain the plant's essential oil. The other varieties have oil glands, but rather than being translucent they are the color of rust and look like spots.

The buds and flowers contain the chief active healing ingredient of St. John's Wort. If you rub the buds and flowers between your fingers a deep, wine-red pigment will be released. It is this secretion that contains the active chemical constituent called hypericin.

During September, and until early October, the flowers produce tiny blackish seeds. The plant dies down in early winter, after the first frosts, and reappears in the spring, shooting up stalkless, short, pale green leaves (with a hint of blue) that grow in pairs opposite each other. Mature plants form branching erect stems when fully

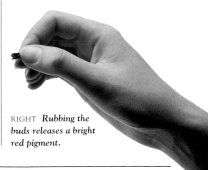

RIGHT **Rubbing the buds releases a bright red pigment.**

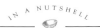
Exploring St. John's Wort

FOUND THROUGHOUT THE WORLD, *in a wide range of habitats, St. John's Wort appears to thrive in fertile, well-drained soil, with plentiful water in late spring and summer.*

WHERE TO FIND ST. JOHN'S WORT

The plant is native to all parts of Britain and the majority of mainland Europe, western Asia, and North Africa, growing prolifically in all these areas. St. John's Wort has been introduced to other countries over the last 200 years and now grows wild in parts of the United States, notably in the temperate western regions from the Pacific Northwest to Northern California, and in central Nevada. It is also to be found in Australia and Canada, the latter mainly in Quebec and Ontario.

BELOW **St. John's Wort grows in the prairie states of the US.**

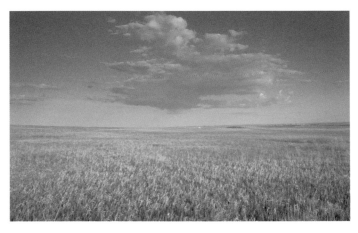

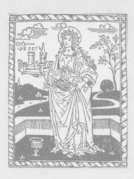

A MEDIEVAL SAYING

St. John's Wort doth charm
all witches away

If gathered at midnight on
the saint's holy day.

Any devils and witches have
no power to harm

Those that gather the plant
for a charm.

LEFT *Detail from a manuscript showing a woman gathering herbs, dated c.1400 CE*

COMMERCIAL GROWERS

The main areas where St. John's Wort is cultivated commercially are the northwestern states and especially the prairie states of the United States. It is also farmed in Canada, Australia, and Germany.

SOIL REQUIREMENTS

St. John's Wort is a hardy plant able to proliferate at speed in the right conditions. In the United States and Australia, where it is not native, it is now subject to statutory weed control – or at least noted as a widespread nuisance by those who don't use it medicinally. St. John's Wort prefers well-drained to dry soil and is often found either where the soil has recently been disturbed or in chalky, sandy, or very light soils. It performs best on neutral to acid soils, but doesn't do well on alkaline types. However, it can thrive in sun or partial shade.

Because it grows well on non-alkaline soils, St. John's Wort is easy to cultivate commercially. This is mainly done in the dominant farming areas of the United States, where the wide open, easily managed lands of the prairies (loam- or gravel-based soils) need little or no fertilization.

RIGHT *Flowers and leaves of St. John's Wort.*

A history of healing

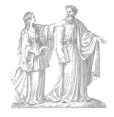

ABOVE **Druids used the herb in their rites.**

ST. JOHN'S WORT *has a 2,400-year history of recorded use, from ancient civilizations in Greece, through pagan Europe and the Middle Ages, to the modern day. After the 1930s it faded from popularity, but it is now recognized as one of the most effective of the healing herbs, and is in the process of regaining its traditional status.*

The name St. John probably refers to John the Baptist, whom tradition said was born on the summer solstice. It was claimed that the red spots visible on the underside of some of the herb's leaves symbolized the blood of St. John, who was beheaded by Herod. However, being blood red it also symbolized healing. Traditionally the flowers were put under the pillow on St. John's Eve in the belief that the saint would appear in a dream to give his blessing – and ensure that the sleeper would not die during the following 12 months – a significant "safeguard" during days when life was cheap and plague epidemics rife.

BELOW **Leaves were left under the pillow on St. John's Eve.**

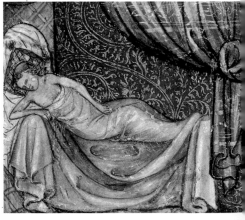

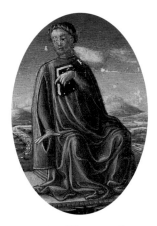

ABOVE *The renowned Greek herbalist Pliny used St. John's Wort.*

However, the plant can be traced back still further. Because its first summer flowers appear near or even on the summer solstice, it was always an icon of sun worshippers, used in solstice rites by the Druids, the Celts and the Saxons, and for centuries the Romans burned it in bonfires as part of their celebration of Midsummer's Day.

The renowned Greek herbalists of the 1st century CE – Pliny, Discorides, and Hippocrates – all used this herb, while the ancient Greek scholar, Galen, described it as "the antidote to intestinal worms."

NAMES AND FOLKLORE

The Greek herbalists' varied uses for St. John's Wort must in part have given rise to the Greek roots that are apparent in its Latin names. *Hypereikon* is Greek for "above" (*hyper*) and "picture" (*eikon*) which, some authorities suggest, explains the prominent role it was given in decorating people's homes during celebrations.

The Latin word *perforatum* literally describes the tiny oil gland perforations on the back of the leaf. Medieval tales embellish this description by adding that the leaves were put into the undergarments of virgins to protect their chastity. The marks on the leaves were said to have been made by the Devil as he tried to "enter" the virgins.

Another ancient name for St. John's Wort was *Fuga Daemonum*, meaning "Scare Devil," another indication that it was thought to drive out demons. It was also believed that if you stepped on the plant at twilight, you might be carried off on a magic horse and not be returned until daybreak.

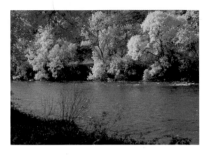

ABOVE *St. John's Wort grows profusely around the Klamath River in California.*

RECENT HISTORY

Other common names for St. John's Wort include Amber (no doubt from the color of the oil) and, in the United States, Klamath weed, because it naturalized around the Klamath River in California. European settlers introduced St. John's Wort to America in the late 18th century, and its cultivation soon became widespread. Its importance in the New World is attested by its appearance in *King's American Dispensatory*, an important work first published in 1898. Written by H. Felter and J. Lloyd, this volume became a classic of herbal medicine and is still consulted today. It lists many uses for St. John's Wort, ranging from colds to insanity, with an emphasis on how the herb specializes in curing nervous and respiratory illnesses.

From the early 1900s, St. John's Wort has been used to help in the treatment of degenerative nerve conditions such as multiple sclerosis, while recent research has suggested that the herb can help to combat alcoholism.

BELOW *A modern herbalist at work.*

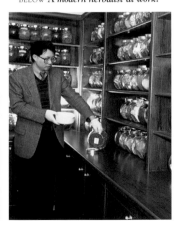

LEFT *The oil derived from St. John's Wort has a distinctive amber color.*

TRADITIONAL APPLICATIONS

King's American Dispensatory listed the following applications for St. John's Wort. Many of them have been confirmed since by modern herbalists, and some (notably depression) have been proven by scientific research:

INTERNAL

- Anemia • Bedwetting
- Blood purifier • Burns
- Congestion • Colds
- Diarrhea • Digestive stimulant • Dysentery
- Headaches • Insomnia
- Jaundice • Mania, hysteria, and madness
- Nerve conditions, including depression and stress reactions
- Neuralgia and shingles
- Rheumatic aches and pains • Syphilis
- Phlebitis • Urinary problems: increases output and eases general bladder ailments
- Uterine cramping
- Worms
- Wound healing

EXTERNAL

- Bruises • Burns, scalds, and blisters
- Mastitis • Neuralgia and shingles
- Sensitive skin problems
- Sores (all types)
- Ulcers • Wounds

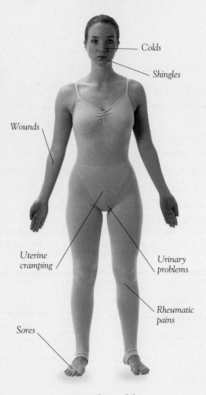

Colds

Shingles

Wounds

Uterine cramping

Urinary problems

Rheumatic pains

Sores

ABOVE *Some of the problems that St. John's Wort can treat.*

13

Anatomy of St. John's Wort

ONLY THE AERIAL PARTS *of St. John's Wort are used – the buds, flowers, and leaves, along with the stalks attached to these parts. Unlike many herbs, the root is not used because it doesn't contain any detectable healing constituents.*

BUDS AND FLOWERS

The buds form a small and neat oval shape, with delicate green sepals like a candle holder. The star-shaped, golden yellow flowers cluster together like blossom on branched stems. They are about 1in (2.5cm) across and have tiny faint black margins along the petals. When you crush the flowers and buds, they leave a magnificent deep magenta stain.

Chemical constituents

A class of naturally occurring plant chemicals called naphthodianthrones (sometimes known as dianthrones) contain the two important healing substances hypericin and pseudohypericin, which are found mainly in the buds and flowers of the herb.

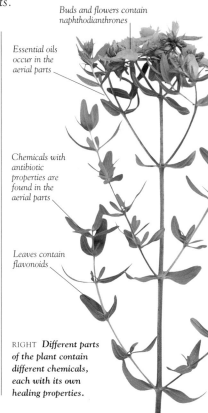

Buds and flowers contain naphthodianthrones

Essential oils occur in the aerial parts

Chemicals with antibiotic properties are found in the aerial parts

Leaves contain flavonoids

RIGHT **Different parts of the plant contain different chemicals, each with its own healing properties.**

SHELF LIFE
dried buds and flowers last
6–9 months;
fresh buds and flowers last
3 days for maximum potency.

LEAVES AND STEMS

The stems are rigid (two-sided) but otherwise smooth. They hold themselves erect and are increasingly branched toward the top of the plant. Each branch grows in a different direction (alternately) for maximum exposure to light. The pale green leaves are small, only 1in (2.5cm) in length, and are oblong and smooth (they have no "teeth"). They have tiny translucent gland sacs (perforations) on the underside of their leaves.

ST. JOHN'S BLOOD

The faint black marks on the leaves of this herb were said to be a symbol of the beheading of St. John the Baptist at the cruel insistence of Herod's daughter, Salome. If the blossoms are put in oil and left to infuse in the sun, the oil gradually becomes a rich red. Traditionally, this was known as St. John's blood.

Chemical constituents

The flavonoids in the leaves and stems contain many derivatives – quercetin, hyperoside, isoquercitrin, rutin, lureolin, and amentoflavone – with the last of these being responsible for St. John's Wort's key antidepressant action.

There are other important chemicals that can be found throughout the aerial parts of the plant: these include phloroglucinols and their derivatives hyperforin, adhyperforin, and hyperside, all of which contain major antibiotic properties.

Essential oils are also present in the leaves and stems: these include monoterpenes and sesquiterpenes, which are known to have sedative properties.

SHELF LIFE
whole dried leaves and stems
last 6–12 months; dried last
6–9 months;
fresh leaves and stems last
3 days for maximum potency.

St. John's Wort in action

ST. JOHN'S WORT IS *known to treat a wide and varied range of disorders, utilizing only the aerial parts of the plant for both internal and external use.*

HOW ST. JOHN'S WORT CAN HELP

🌿 Eases post-surgery swelling, bruises, sprains, muscle aches, toothache (including tooth removal and abscesses), cuts, trapped nerves, neuralgia, sciatica, and fibrositis.

BELOW *St. John's Wort eases swelling to bruises and sprains.*

🌿 Helps in the treatment of many skin disorders including psoriasis, eczema, and warts.

🌿 Useful for kidney and bladder complaints, including incontinence.

🌿 Treats a wide range of viral, bacterial, and microbial invasions and many other disorders that are usually treated by antibiotics, especially stomach and gastrointestinal complaints.

🌿 St. John's Wort is also effective against diarrhea and viral infections like herpes simplex and influenza.

🌿 Soothes and heals inflamed tissue and reduces pain, thus making the herb effective in cases of rheumatism and arthritis and many other similar conditions. St. John's Wort can appropriately be used internally or externally in order to ease the severity of these complaints.

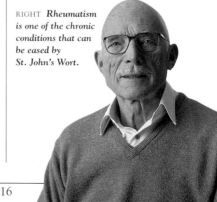

RIGHT *Rheumatism is one of the chronic conditions that can be eased by St. John's Wort.*

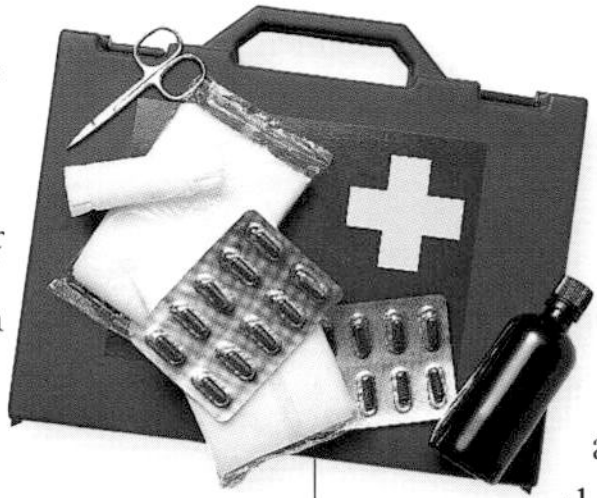

RIGHT ***St. John's Wort is a useful addition to every first aid box.***

- Aids the relief of lung problems such as congestion and chronic catarrh.
- Helpful during the menopause and for postmenopausal women.
- Can help to treat dysentery and parasitic worm infestations.
- Helps the liver to recover from jaundice, hepatitis, inflammation of the liver, and similar conditions, as well as gall bladder complaints and related digestive disorders.
- Treats a range of nerve- and brain-related disorders, from anxiety to sleep disorders such as insomnia, early morning waking, and oversleeping. Also eases some psychological disturbances, including depression, nervous excitement, some tension headaches, premenstrual syndrome, menopausal symptoms, impaired memory, and dyslexia.
- The generalized wound-healing abilities of St. John's Wort make it ideal for the first-aid kit for use on burns, chapped skin, frostbite, insect bites, and sunburn.

It was said that the Christian Crusaders used the flowers and leaves of St. John's Wort crushed into lard as poultices to heal their sword wounds.

HOW ST. JOHN'S WORT AFFECTS THE BODY

- Antidepressant (helps to change mood).
- Antioxidant (prevents free radicals causing damage to cells – see page 56).
- Antiviral (effective against disease-carrying viruses).
- Anti-inflammatory (reduces inflammation).
- Anti-microbial (disarms microbes).
- Analgesic (pain relief).
- Antispasmodic (relaxes muscular contractions).
- Aromatic (digestive).
- Astringent (tones and heals).
- Expectorant (provokes the release of mucus).
- Nervine (feeds and calms the nervous system).
- Hepatic (favorably influences the liver and gall bladder).

EFFECTS

The nervous system is affected by St. John's Wort in many ways. One of these is to increase "theta waves" in the brain during waking hours. Theta waves usually occur only during sleep, deep meditation, moments of serene pleasure, and heightened creative activity. The herb may also help to sharpen perception and clarify the thinking process, improving the speed and ability with which the brain processes information and the memory retains it.

St. John's Wort also helps to combat depression, including Seasonal Affective Disorder (SAD). It is believed that the herb does this by increasing the amount of three particular chemicals in the brain, collectively called neurotransmitters, which serve to pass on certain messages – these chemicals are serotonin, norepinephrine, and dopamine. **Serotonin** is mood enhancing – low levels are directly responsible for feelings of depression; **norepinephrine** is responsible for energy and alertness; and **dopamine** is a general "feel good" brain chemical.

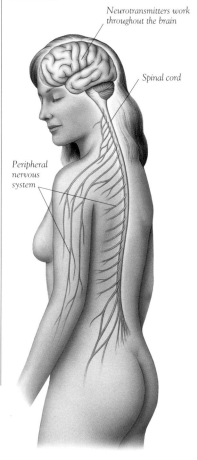

Neurotransmitters work throughout the brain

Spinal cord

Peripheral nervous system

RIGHT *St. John's Wort is thought to affect both the brain's activity and the nervous system.*

It was originally thought that St. John's Wort increased these key chemicals by inhibiting an enzyme called monoamine oxidase, but this now appears to be incorrect. Today's research speculates that its effectiveness is based on a synergy of interactions, not yet fully understood, that prevents the brain from reabsorbing these neurotransmitters – thus maintaining them at a higher level in the brain. This has a positive effect on the hypothalamus, the region of the brain that controls some important body functions such as thirst, appetite, and body temperature. The hypothalamus is affected by thoughts and feelings, whether they are happy or sad, and so St. John's Wort may have a direct effect on how well the immune system works, preventing it from sending out destructive messages to the cells.

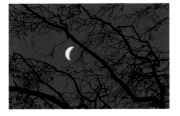

ABOVE *The herb may help treat Seasonal Affective Disorder, which is aggravated by lack of light.*

St. John's Wort has also displayed a wide range of microbial capabilities in fighting many bacteria such as Mycobacterium tuberculosis, Shigella, and E. coli bacteria, plus other strains of bacteria that are highly resistant to antibiotics, for example Staphylococcus aureus, Enterococcus and Pseudomonas aeruginosa. Antibiotic compounds in the herb – hyperforin and novoimanine – kill the bacteria, and stimulate the immune system. St. John's Wort's anti-inflammatory effectiveness stems from its ability to balance the effects of the immune system.

RIGHT *St. John's Wort's antibiotic properties are effective against bacteria.*

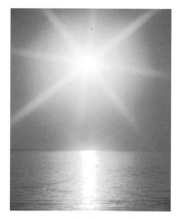

ABOVE *People susceptible to strong sunlight should be especially careful.*

WHEN TO AVOID ST JOHN'S WORT

Phototoxicity

St. John's Wort's most known side effect is "phototoxicity." Light-skinned people in particular may develop a sensitivity to the ultraviolet rays in sunlight, both in the eyes and on the skin, where use of the herb can cause loss of pigmentation or small welts, especially during the summer months. The reason is the interaction of the herb's chemical hypericin with sunlight and oxygen. This occurs because St. John's Wort has the ability to reach the blood and skin without being intercepted and processed by the liver and kidneys. If you find you are susceptible, it's advisable to wear dark glasses and use plenty of suntan lotion – never use sun beds, which often emit large amounts of ultraviolet light.

Other contraindications

❀ Don't take St. John's Wort if you are pregnant or breastfeeding.
❀ Don't take St. John's Wort while using amino-acid supplements.

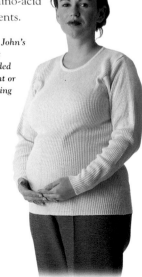

RIGHT *St. John's Wort is not recommended for pregnant or breast-feeding women.*

✤ Don't take St. John's Wort with chronic liver and kidney disease unless you are under direct medical supervision because, if the herb behaves in a toxic fashion, these organs appear to be unable to detoxify accumulations. Liver and kidney cleansing programs will help (see pages 22–3).

✤ Don't take St. John's Wort if you have an estrogen-driven cancer of the reproductive system such as breast or ovarian cancer.

✤ Don't mix St. John's Wort with antidepressant drugs (especially any type containing monoamine oxidase, for example diet pills and nasal sprays).

✤ Don't take St. John's Wort with the herb Yohimbe, which also contains monoamine oxidase.

✤ Don't use the herb with drugs aimed at decreasing dopaminergic activity (see page 18) or which are treating any kind of mental disorder.

> **CAUTION**
>
> Don't use St. John's Wort if you suffer from manic depression. Indeed, you shouldn't treat serious depression at all yourself. Always seek help in such cases from a qualified professional.

OTHER POSSIBLE SIDE EFFECTS

St. John's Wort can produce other, less common side effects in some people. Stop using the herb at once if any of the following symptoms occurs:

✤ Nausea
✤ Fatigue
✤ Anxiety
✤ Disorientation and speech difficulty
✤ Rigidity of neck muscles or contractions of other muscles
✤ Pupil dilation
✤ Sudden rise in blood pressure and/or palpitations
✤ Severe sweating and high fever
✤ Severe headache that worsens on lying down

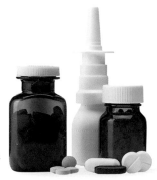

RIGHT **St. John's Wort should not be taken with antidepressant drugs.**

LIVER AND KIDNEY CLEANSING PROGRAM

There is some anxiety among practitioners about using St. John's Wort if you suffer from chronic liver or kidney disease.

However, whatever your situation and state of health, cleansing these organs by an effective method, which does not use the herb, will certainly lead to an improved sense of well-being.

TO MAKE A FRESH "LIVER DRINK"

FOR ONE PERSON

1 or 2 freshly squeezed lemons
1 cup (225ml) apple juice, preferably freshly squeezed
1 cup (225ml) spring water
1 clove fresh garlic (crush before putting into blender)
1 tbsp (15ml) extra virgin olive oil
¼in (5mm) fresh Ginger root (not to be included if your liver feels hot or inflamed)

Consume this drink for one morning on an empty stomach, or for 3–5 consecutive days, during which time you should eat plenty of fresh vegetables, fruit, rice, and other whole foods. Avoid alcohol, tea, coffee, and "junk" foods. Drink copious amounts of spring water.

To make the drink, liquidize the ingredients

RIGHT **Mix apple juice, lemon, Garlic, and Ginger root for a cleansing drink.**

until well blended. Drink slowly. After 15 minutes, drink a cup of hot peppermint tea, followed by some organic apple juice.

You may experience headaches, rashes, sadness, anger, and other unpleasant side effects associated with the shedding of toxins stored in the liver, but these will eventually be replaced by joy and enthusiasm once the cleanse has finished.

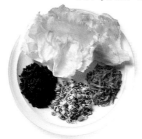

LEFT *For lunch eat a raw salad.*

ONE-DAY "KIDNEY FLUSH"

Choose a day when you can be relaxed and warm. Start the morning by drinking a mixture of the juice of a lemon or lime, 2 US pints (1 liter) of spring water and a pinch of Cayenne. Fifteen minutes later drink a cup of "kidney tea" containing equal parts of Dandelion leaves, Parsley leaves, Uva Ursi leaves, and Corn Silk.

At lunchtime drink diluted fresh raw vegetable juices, or eat a large raw salad made up of ingredients such as sprouted seeds, dandelion leaves, lettuce, grated beets, and grated carrot. For dressings, use olive oil, apple cider vinegar, and lemon juice, with a little Cayenne and black pepper. Drink a cup of barley water 1 hour after your salad.

In total drink 3 cups of kidney tea or 3 cups of barley water. Also try to consume a total of 6–8 US pints (3–4 liters) of spring water.

You may feel cold or experience feelings of weepiness or vulnerability, but these will soon be replaced with calmness and positivity soon after the cleanse has finished.

TO MAKE BARLEY WATER

FOR ONE PERSON

½ cup (100g) whole barley (not pearl barley)
5 cups (1.5 liters) water
¼ cinnamon stick
grated Ginger root, to taste

1 *Put all the ingredients into a pan and bring to a boil.*

2 *Reduce the heat, then simmer for about 20 minutes.*

3 *Strain the mixture into a pitcher, then add fresh lemon juice for extra flavor. Drink 1–3 times daily.*

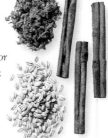

RIGHT **Grated ginger, barley, and cinnamon sticks.**

Energy and emotion

ST. JOHN'S WORT can have a profound effect on mood, enhancing feelings of well-being, reducing fears, and inducing a calming of the spirit.

The bitter taste of the fresh St. John's Wort plant and its subsequent tinctures, infusions, and powders provide a strong hint about its effect in relation to the liver and gall bladder. The taste will immediately activate bile and digestive juices, and the whole effect will be to energize the liver. A stagnant liver can cause a range of emotional states – depression, anger, or sadness – but these can be coaxed to the surface and ultimately lessened as time goes by, resulting in a more positive, lively and excited feeling. It's not a coincidence that the words "life" and "liver" are very similar – they come from the same root.

St. John's Wort also has an astringent taste, which gives clues to effects the herb has on different organs. For example, the kidneys, bladder, and lungs all benefit from it. These organs

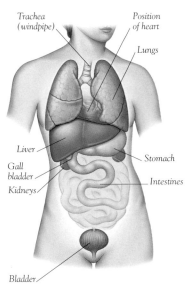

Trachea (windpipe)
Position of heart
Lungs
Liver
Gall bladder
Kidneys
Stomach
Intestines
Bladder

ABOVE *The lungs, stomach, kidneys, and bladder all benefit from the herb's effects.*

gain from the healing, tanning, and drying effect of this astringent quality, and will work better as a result. The emotional effects will be as apparent as the physical ones: as the lungs relax and work better, apprehensions will be lessened; and when the bladder and kidneys work more efficiently, minor fears will fade.

With St. John's Wort, digestion will be increasingly enlivened and will function more harmoniously, assimilating and processing more effectively. This will in turn settle the mind, and the combined effect will be to give you a greater interest in life.

ENERGY AND THE MIND

St. John's Wort invites a deeper state of relaxation, serenity, and contentment. Because it affects the physical and mental state so radically, it is able to flush out "evils" and poisons from the mind, body, and spirit, whenever they appear. The herb gives a sense of confidence and ability, enabling you to enjoy life from a position of calm, with a greater sense of enthusiasm, and vitality.

St. John's Wort banishes negativity and fears, helps you leap over everyday difficulties, and invites lightness and positivity. The herb introduces laughter and relaxation into the life of anyone who uses it.

BELOW *Taking St. John's Wort helps to promote a positive and happy outlook on life.*

FLOWER REMEDIES

St. John's Wort is capable of introducing light and energy into your life on a psychic and emotional level as well as a physical one. It brightens and heals, helping you to glow and radiate. It may help support those who are overstretched in their activities, harnessing their available energy to achieve a more balanced existence.

TO MAKE A FLOWER ESSENCE

STANDARD QUANTITY

Approx. 1½ cups (350ml) each of spring water and brandy, and 3–4 St. John's Wort flowers

1 *Submerge carefully chosen buds and flower heads – freshly picked in the early morning – into a shallow bowl of spring water (use a glass bowl if possible) and place in the sunshine for several hours.*

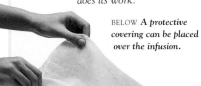

LEFT **The first stage is to infuse the buds and flowers in water in a sunny place.**

If you wish, place a protective covering over the top (freshly washed white muslin is ideal) or leave uncovered while the sun does its work.

BELOW **A protective covering can be placed over the infusion.**

2 *Choose a very sheltered spot and try to ensure you have at least three hours of continuous sun. If the flowers wilt sooner than this, they can be removed earlier.*

3 *Remove the flowers, using a twig to lift them out. Measure the remaining liquid and add an equal measure of brandy to preserve the liquid. Pour the mixture into dark glass bottles and label clearly.*

Recommended dosage

❋ *Adults: 4 drops under the tongue 4 times daily, or every ½ hour in times of crisis. Children: see page 45.*

St. John's Wort radiates bliss and has an immensely protective nature, so people who feel depressed or negative in any way will really benefit from this flower essence.

LEFT *When ready, the infusion is poured into dark glass bottles.*

CASE STUDY: DEPRESSION

John had suffered from depression since childhood. It worsened during puberty but stabilized in adulthood. Shy, introverted, and incommunicative, even with his close family, John heard about St. John's Wort's antidepressant qualities and, having long before given up on proprietary drugs, he consulted a herbalist. He began with 1 tsp (5ml) of tincture three times daily – and on the third day phoned the clinic to say he felt like a different person. For the first time he could remember, he was having warm and meaningful conversations with his family. He noticed other changes – like enthusiasm for work and a completely fresh awareness of colors. John remained in touch with his herbal practitioner over the next few months to monitor his progress with the herb.

PLANT SPIRIT ENERGIES

The spirit of the plant is different to a flower essence, which is connected principally with its flowering aspect. The plant's spirit enables every part of it to share its energy and properties with us. The ability of St. John's Wort to thrive and colonize almost anywhere, while giving light and serenity, gives us a clue to its spirit. Earthy yet illuminating, it can take us from some very primitive emotional states or mental processes to some extremely meditative and joyful ones.

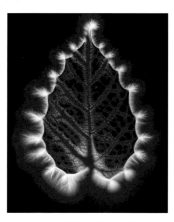

ABOVE *Kirlian photography can capture the spirit energy of a plant.*

Growing, harvesting, and processing

St. John's Wort is not difficult to grow as long as you provide soil with adequate drainage. It looks beautiful in the garden and will provide an abundance of flowers and leaves for healing.

GROWING ST. JOHN'S WORT

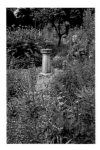

ABOVE **The plant is an attractive addition to any garden.**

St. John's Wort will grow almost anywhere in temperate regions. It is a very versatile plant and thrives in poor soil, but it is also at home in good-quality tilth (see page 9). Although it prefers full sun, the herb will also grow in shaded areas. It doesn't like too much water and therefore soil with good drainage is preferable. The best time to plant St. John's Wort is late fall or early spring. It can easily be grown from seed or runners, and can be transplanted without difficulty.

Homegrown The fact that this plant grows wild in so many places throughout the temperate world is an indication of how easy it is to cultivate at home. For planting, select an area of your garden that has poor to average soil and has been well dug. The bed should be about 3ft (1m) wide and 1ft (30cm) deep.

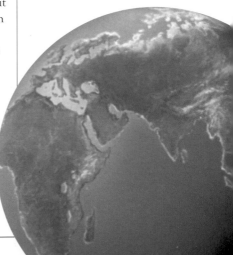

Scatter the seeds on the prepared ground, give them some water, and let nature do its work. The secret to the successful propagation of St. John's Wort is to ignore it as much as possible: it doesn't need fertilizing, feeding, or pruning. However, if there is a drought, keep it watered, but not saturated, and cover it if there is likely to be an overnight frost.

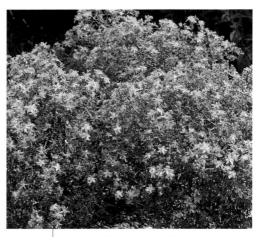

ABOVE *The best time to harvest is just after the plant has started to bloom.*

HARVESTING

Commercial The aerial parts of St. John's Wort are collected between mid-June and late August in colder areas, but always when the plant is just beginning to bloom (20–50% in flower), when the hypericin content is at its highest. From 75% bloom to the post-flowering stage the hypericin content drops off dramatically, and drying

becomes much more difficult. Analysis of plant chemistry levels using "gas chromatography" now provides a scientific approach to optimum harvesting time, but this is not necessary if the aforementioned "bloom test" is applied.

Commercial growers cut off the top 6–10in (15–25cm) of the leafy stem, buds, and flowers, using heavy machinery and collecting bins. On some herb farms they are harvested by hand, using machete knives. The roots are left intact so that new foliage will return the following spring.

LEFT *St. John's Wort thrives across most of the temperate regions of the globe.*

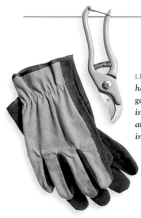

LEFT *The herb can be gathered in small amounts in the wild.*

Gathering the wild herb When picking St. John's Wort in the wild, it's important never to take more than a third or so of any plant family or colony, in order to leave plenty of flowers to provide seed for next year. Exceptions to this rule are in areas of the United States and Australia because the herb is so invasive there.

PROCESSING

Commercial Once the aerial parts of the plant are cut and collected, they are best dried in the shade for some time: direct sunlight will rapidly strip the vital chemistries from the plant. With some commercial crops, however, full sun is allowed for between 3 and 5 hours (according to the sun's intensity), to allow the herb to wilt. Drying then continues in the shade on slatted racks or in a commercial drier. The maximum moisture content should be no more than 5–8% at the end of the drying process.

After being fully dried, the raw material of dried leaves, buds, and flowers is stored in a dry, covered area with adequate airflow, and "turned" on a daily basis. The dried herbs are then chopped into ½–1in (1–2.5cm) segments. Checks are made to ensure that no molds have occurred before packing. The herb is stored in burlap bags with good air circulation, ready for sending to commercial processors by truck or plane. Some commercial farms process their herbs on site, and make fresh products such as tinctures or cold-pressed oils.

LEFT *When picking wild flowers, leave two thirds to grow for the following year.*

Home processing

As with the commercial process, you should give the aerial parts of the plant a few hours of direct sunlight, by which time they will have wilted – and any visiting bugs that were in them should

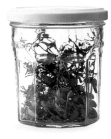

ABOVE **When they are dry, put the plants in a glass jar.**

have crawled away. Shake all the pieces of the gathered plant to make sure that any remaining bugs are dislodged.

Place the wilted plants in brown paper bags and hang them in a very dry, temperate place. You can tell when the plants are dry because they will no longer be limp and will crumble easily when touched.

When you feel they are dry enough, put the contents in a glass jar, cover with an airtight lid, then leave the jar in the sunshine. If water droplets appear on the insides of the jar, there is still some moisture in the plant material and therefore a risk of spoilage, so you should remove the contents from the jar and dry them for a while longer, before storing in a dry, dark place.

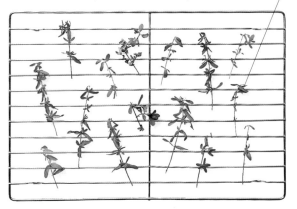

BELOW **Late summer leaves and tiny buds being dried after the second harvest of the season.**

Wilted plants are well spaced

Preparations for internal use

ABOVE **Cold-pressed oil, for most uses.**

ST. JOHN'S WORT *can be taken internally in the form of tincture, infusion, or capsule. Cold-pressed oil and fresh juice can be used internally as well as externally, depending on the conditions being treated.*

ST. JOHN'S WORT TINCTURE

In this form the herb is concentrated yet liquid. It's normally sold in dark blue or brown glass bottles, but for larger amounts it can be stored in opaque plastic containers for a limited amount of time. Whether your tincture is bought or homemade, it's handy to keep some in the smaller "dropper" bottles for your purse, briefcase, or pocket to make dosing easier.

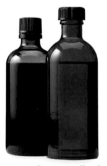

ABOVE **Commercially, the tincture is sold in dark glass bottles.**

Use fresh herbs if possible because some of the hypericin and other chemical components are lost during the drying process. If you cannot get the fresh herb, however, the dried herb will still be adequate.

St. John's Wort tincture is made by soaking the chopped or shredded aerial parts – leaves, stalks, buds, and flowers – in alcohol and water. It's better to extract it this way because alcohol and water retain some of the wide range of chemical constituents that heal the body. It's particularly

LEFT **You can use fresh or dried St. John's Wort to make a tincture.**

RIGHT *Herbalists occasionally make tinctures according to the moon's cycle.*

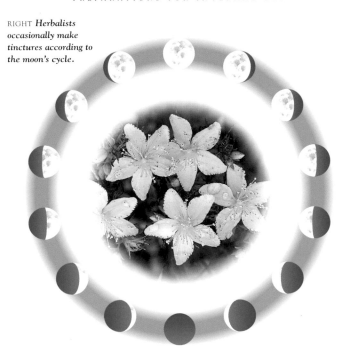

important when using fresh herbs, which are more likely to be infested with opportunistic fungi and bacteria. Pouring alcohol onto your herbs kills any germs, and water can be added later when they have been destroyed.

Commercially, St. John's Wort tincture is made with good quality, high percentage alcohol, with a total mix of 45% alcohol to 55% water. If you are making

tincture at home, you can use vodka (see page 34).

The tincturing process takes a minimum of 14 days, but you can leave it for up to four weeks. Some herbalists like to utilize the gravitational waxing and waning of the moon during the process. You make the tincture at the time of the new moon, and then strain and bottle it at the full moon.

TO MAKE A ROOT TINCTURE

STANDARD QUANTITY

As a rough guide, use 4–5½ cups (225–310g) of fresh herb
chopped into small pieces, or bought shredded, to
2 US pints (1 liter) of alcohol and water mixture.

1 *Place the fresh or dried St. John's Wort leaves, buds, and flowers in a liquidizer or food processor and cover with vodka; 37–45% proof vodka is standard, but a higher proof (70–80%) is always better. Liquidize the contents – they will mix fairly easily, because the*

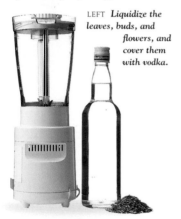

LEFT **Liquidize the leaves, buds, and flowers, and cover them with vodka.**

NOTE

Always clean your utensils before
use in boiling water, and for best
results add one or two drops of
essential oil such as lavender,
thyme, or tea tree to the water.

flowers, leaves, and buds are flexible and delicate in nature. When blended, pour into a dark glass jar or preserving jar, shake well, and label carefully. Store for two days, shaking the jar each day to help the extraction process.

2 *After two days, add water to the mixture. If you have used standard proof alcohol and dried herbs, you need to add only 20% of water to the total quantity of liquidized mash. If you have used higher proof alcohol and dried herbs, then instead you'll need to add 50–60% water to the mash. However, if you have used fresh herbs, the higher moisture content means you will need to add only about 10% water.*

3 *Strain the tincture through a jelly bag, preferably overnight, until you have the very last drop of liquid. For best results use a wine press instead.*

4 *Pour the thick liquid into dark glass jars, label clearly, and store in a dark place. For personal use, decant into smaller 2fl oz (50ml) tincture bottles.*

Recommended dosage

❋ **Everyday use** *Adults should take ½ tsp (2.5ml) of tincture 2–3 times a day, diluted in 5 tsp (25ml) of water or fruit juice. Double this dose can be taken where speed of treatment is an important factor. Children over 12 years of age can take the adult dose but only once daily; children under 12 years should only take St. John's Wort under the guidance of a suitably qualified herbalist or medical practitioner (see page 45).*

❋ **Long-term use** *This herb can be taken safely for months or even years, especially if it's being used to treat depression over extended periods of time. Adult dose: 40 drops, 2–3 times daily. Children: over 12 years old, the adult dose of 40 drops but only 1–3 times daily; for children under 12 years, see page 45.*

❋ **Periodic use** *Some people like to take St. John's Wort for a few weeks and then have a break from it for a similar period. This routine can help to keep the brain chemicals balanced without the user having to take the herb daily. The dosages to be taken during the periods of use are the same as for long-term use.*

REMOVING THE ALCOHOL

Diabetics may not wish to ingest the small amount of alcohol contained in the tincture. You can reduce it by adding a little boiling water to the dose and leaving it to stand for about 5 minutes while evaporation takes place; around 98.5% of the alcohol will "burn off."

Teetotallers who want to avoid alcohol altogether can replace the vodka with apple cider vinegar. Recovering alcoholics may be better off taking St. John's Wort Extraction Capsules (see page 37) or in oil form (see page 38).

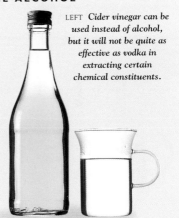

LEFT **Cider vinegar can be used instead of alcohol, but it will not be quite as effective as vodka in extracting certain chemical constituents.**

ST. JOHN'S WORT INFUSION

Making St. John's Wort infusion isn't usually recommended, because water alone fails to release all of the important chemical components, especially those used to treat depression. Nevertheless, infusions have their uses, and are easier and quicker to make than tinctures. They are generally employed to help a wide range of non-depressive disorders that include bedwetting, bladder infection, and liver problems.

TO MAKE AN INFUSION

STANDARD QUANTITY

1 tsp (2–3g) dried herb or 2 tsp (4–6g) fresh herb to 1 cup (250ml) water

or

1oz (25g) dried herb or 1¼oz (35g) fresh herb to 2 cups (500ml) water

1 Put the herb in a tea sock and place in a cup or teapot. Pour on boiling water and leave to stand for 7–10 minutes. (You can also use a special teapot infuser, or a coffee pot with a plunger.)

2 Remove the tea sock and, if desired, add half a teaspoon of organic, cold-pressed honey (although it's best without added sweetness).

Recommended dosage

❋ Adults: 2 cups daily – in total 500ml per day. Children: over 12 years old, adult dose; younger than 12, see page 45.

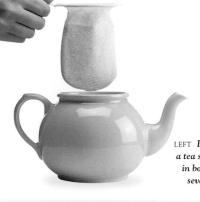

LEFT **Put the herb into a tea sock and steep it in boiling water for several minutes.**

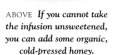

ABOVE **If you cannot take the infusion unsweetened, you can add some organic, cold-pressed honey.**

CAPSULES

There is a commercial process called "alcoholic extraction LI160," which starts in a similar way to tincturing. Alcohol is used to dissolve the useful chemicals before being evaporated off. Each extract is then tested and adjusted so that the strength is uniform. The powdered extracts are then made into capsules or tablets. This is the best way for recovering alcoholics to take St. John's Wort because there is no alcohol content (see also page 35).

St. John's Wort capsules can also be made simply by using powdered herb.

ABOVE *You can buy size 00 vegetable capsules from a herbalist.*

TO MAKE CAPSULES

STANDARD QUANTITY

Approximately 250–300mg of powdered herb fits into a size 00 capsule.

1 *Put a little dried, finely powdered St. John's Wort in a saucer and open up the ends of a capsule.*

2 *Using the ends as shovels, push them together until they are full (one end will have more herb than the other). Join the two ends carefully so that you do not lose any of the powder while you do so.*

Recommended dosage

❋ **Powdered capsule** *Adults: a 300mg strength capsule three-times daily. Children: over 12 years old, adult dose; younger than 12, see page 45.*

❋ **Alcohol extraction capsule** *Adults: a 300mg strength capsule three times daily. Children: over 12 years old, adult dose; younger than 12, see page 45.*

BELOW *Scoop the powdered herb into each end of an opened capsule.*

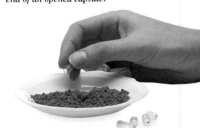

Preparations for external use

ST. JOHN'S WORT *is very effective when used externally on bites, cuts, wounds, bruises, and various skin diseases and conditions. It also helps to relieve general pain, stiffness, and impairment of nerves and muscles.*

St. John's Wort's powerful chemistry goes to work immediately at the site of the problem, in many instances providing rapid relief or cure.

ST. JOHN'S WORT JUICE

You can express the juice from the fresh aerial parts of the herb using a vegetable or fruit juice extractor (not a liquidizer). Take ½ tsp (2.5ml) 3 times daily internally. You can also apply it externally to affected areas with cotton wool. Let it dry freely and repeat when necessary.

CAUTION

The essential oil is for external use only, applied round the edges of the inflammation. Do not use on broken skin or pulse points.

ST. JOHN'S WORT ESSENTIAL OIL

The essential oil of St. John's Wort is pressed from the leaves, buds, and flowers.
Dosage: A total of 5 drops daily, or more with the guidance of a herbalist or aromatherapist. Dilute the drops in a little jojoba oil to avoid skin irritation. Jojoba is a natural sunscreen with a factor of 16, and is absorbed efficiently into the skin without becoming rancid.

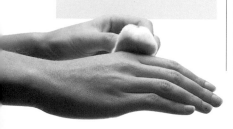

LEFT *St. John's Wort juice is applied to cuts and wounds with cotton wool.*

ST. JOHN'S WORT POULTICE

This is an ideal treatment for nerve or muscle pain. Newly flowering St. John's Wort should be used, preferably with more closed buds than open flowers. The bunch will also have a few leaves and stalks if you pick 2–3in (5–8cm) above the ground; do not discard these but use them too.

TO MAKE A POULTICE

STANDARD QUANTITY

There is no specific requirement on herb quantity, it really depends of the size of body area you wish to treat. Use enough chopped fresh herb to cover the body area affected, and enough water to cover the herb in the pan.

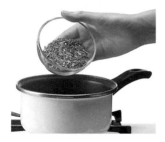

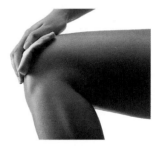

1 *Place the chopped herb in a saucepan and cover with filtered or spring water. Bring to a boil, then simmer for two minutes. Strain and squeeze out the excess liquid.*

2 *Rub some olive oil (or any other suitable pure vegetable oil) onto the affected area – this prevents the hot herb from sticking to the skin.*

3 *Squeeze the hot, damp mixture together onto a poultice (a large plaster or piece of thin gauze) and press onto the affected area. If possible, secure the poultice in place with plastic wrap; this will also help to retain the heat.*

4 *Leave for 2–3 hours and reapply with more hot poultice if necessary. Repeat the process as often as required.*

ST. JOHN'S WORT OINTMENT AND CREAM

These are both effective for bites, cuts, wounds, dry eczema, and psoriasis. Ointments aren't appropriate for hot, wet, oozing conditions because the oil and wax mixture tends to heat up rather than cool down. For these conditions, a cream would be better or you can simply sprinkle dry St. John's Wort powder directly onto the affected area, or mix it with a "carrier" of aloe vera gel.

TO MAKE A CREAM

STANDARD QUANTITY

2¼oz (60g) jar of unscented cold cream to 1 tsp (5ml) St. John's Wort essential oil (see page 38).

Scoop out 1 tablespoonful of cream and discard; stir the oil into the remaining cream.

LEFT **Mix the oil into the cream until you have a smooth consistency.**

TO MAKE AN OINTMENT

STANDARD QUANTITY

1¾ cups (425ml) cold-pressed extra virgin olive oil
6 cups (350g) dried, powdered herbs
2oz (50g) beeswax.

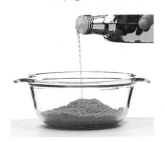

1 *Pour the olive oil onto the powdered herbs and mix together.*

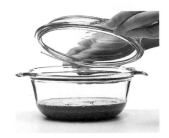

2 *Place in a closed container (ovenproof if you are using the oven method) and either put into an oven preheated to 100°F (38°C) for two hours, or stand in the sun or other warm spot for a week.*

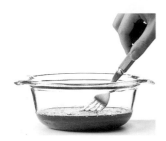

3 During the allotted time, occasionally stir the mixture with a sterilized fork.

4 On completion of slow cooking or soaking, strain the mixture through a large plastic or stainless steel colander lined with muslin, or use a jelly bag and hang it up to drip overnight. If you have used the oven method, reheat the mixture at the same temperature before straining.

5 Finally, melt 2oz (50g) of beeswax over a very low heat in a double boiler or heavy-bottomed pan, then add the herbal olive oil saturate. Put a little of the mixture into a glass jar to check for consistency (it shouldn't be too liquid when cold), before pouring it into dark glass jars. Label clearly.

RIGHT **The mixture is strained through a piece of muslin.**

ST. JOHN'S WORT COLD-PRESSED OIL

Not to be confused with essential oil (see page 38), this ancient method of extracting St. John's Wort's vital plant chemistry is effective, and the resultant rust-red oil can be used internally as well as externally. Sunlight encourages the herb to release its active ingredients and is less harmful than heating the herb. This takes time, so you should allow several weeks to complete the process.

INCREASING THE POTENCY

If you still have some St. John's Wort in flower when you have made the oil, you can add new, fresh herbs to the strained oil, to make it stronger and more effective. Because cold-pressed oil can be used internally as well as on the skin, it's important to use a good quality organic virgin olive oil. This ensures no rancidity, no pesticides, no chemicals used for ripening the olives, and no preservatives.

LEFT **Good quality organic olive oil is ideal to blend with St. John's Wort.**

TO MAKE COLD-PRESSED OIL

STANDARD QUANTITY

Use chopped fresh herb and cold-pressed extra virgin olive oil. A good standard would be to put enough chopped herb into a clean glass jar so that it is three-quarters full, then top up with olive oil.

1 *Shake the plant well to remove any visiting insects.*

2 *Place the freshly picked buds and flowers, along with a few leaves, in a preserving jar. Pack the herbs in as tightly as you can, because this will make a stronger, more concentrated oil.*

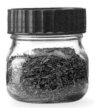

Recommended dosage

❧ *External use: apply liberally and as often as you can until the symptoms ease.*
❧ *Internal use: adults, 1 teaspoonful 3 times a day; children over 12 years old, adult dose; younger than 12, see page 45.*

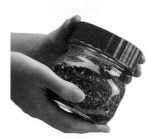

3 Add sufficient olive oil to cover the
herbs, then put on the lid and shake
well. Don't let the herbs oxidize (turn
brown) by letting them protrude above
the level of the oil. Eventually the herbs
will subside well below the surface of the
oil. Shaking as often as possible will help
this process.

4 Place the jar in a warm, sunny
position such as on a window sill or in
a greenhouse. Leave for a minimum of
two weeks, although there's no strict time
limit on the "warming phase" with cold-
pressed oil. I've left the mixture for three
months and found that the oil comes to no
harm as long as it is shaken daily,
especially at the beginning.

RIGHT **The herbs
and oil must be left
in a sunny place.**

5 Strain the
herb and oil
mixture through
a jelly bag or, if
possible, through
a wine press. If
using a jelly
bag, leave it
overnight, then
thoroughly
squeeze any
remaining oil
from the bag.

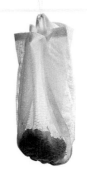

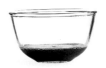

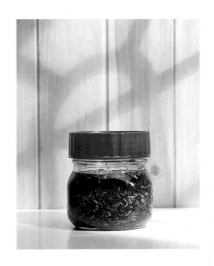

Natural medicine for everyone

ALTHOUGH IN SOME WAYS St. John's Wort is almost a "wonder herb," it isn't applicable to every condition – and care must always be taken with certain groups of people, particularly when the herb is used internally.

PREGNANCY

The internal use of St. John's Wort isn't advised during pregnancy, nor the use of essential oils externally. Research has shown that the herb can cause uterine contractions – indeed Native Americans traditionally used it, along with other herbs, as an abortive. Current research is looking at whether it can also cause cell mutation and, as a result, fetal abnormalities.

LEFT *St. John's Wort should not be taken internally in pregnancy.*

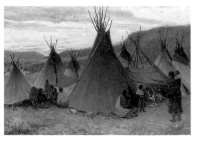

ABOVE *Native Americans used St. John's Wort to induce abortions.*

The use of any antidepressant is questionable during pregnancy, especially in the last three months, due to their effect on the fetus's brain and nervous system. However, minute quantities of St. John's Wort consumed inadvertently should cause no harm.

For the same reasons the use of St. John's Wort is not advised during breastfeeding.

CHILDREN

External use of St. John's Wort cold-pressed oil (or the cream or fresh poultice) is quite safe for children, and they usually love its soothing effect. Internal use for children must be at the discretion of a herbal practitioner, who will employ the correct dosage for their age. Some experts nevertheless suggest that children under the age of 12 shouldn't take St. John's Wort – and never without close medical supervision.

CASE STUDY: TEETH

Ten-year-old Daisy had "crowded teeth" and she needed to have two extracted. An abscess in the same area was giving her additional pain.

Her mother knew about the pain-relieving qualities of St. John's Wort and bought some just before the extraction, putting some on the abscess and taking the bottle to the clinic.

Afterwards she rubbed some more onto Daisy's gums – which were still numb from the anaesthetic – and repeated this hourly until bedtime. Daisy experienced no pain, the abscess subsided, and the gum healed over fast. The dentist was impressed.

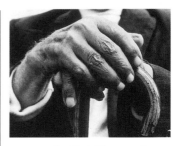

ABOVE *St. John's Wort can relieve psychological, skin, and rheumatic problems in the elderly.*

ELDERLY PEOPLE

St. John's Wort is a very useful herb when administered internally for elderly people, who can easily become depressed by their lack of mobility, by physical disorders (including circulatory conditions), and by psychological problems such as loneliness. They are often given drugs to alleviate these and other problems, but the side effects can be unwelcome.

Elderly people should consult a qualified herbalist before using St. John's Wort internally, but it is unnecessary for external use. Used externally, St. John's Wort can be invaluable for treating bed sores, leg ulcers, and slow-healing wounds or burns, all of which are prevalent among older people who become immobile.

Herbal combinations

HERBAL COMBINATIONS *are used where the effect of a single herb needs to be helped in a particular way. However, if you are pregnant, breastfeeding, or have a serious medical condition, you should consult your doctor or another qualified practitioner first.*

BLADDER AND KIDNEY WEAKNESS

This formula made as a tincture can be used for generalized maintenance. It can also be used for temporary and emotionally based incontinence, where there is infection or other causes.

CAUTION

Don't use any of the complementary formulas during pregnancy or breastfeeding (*see pages 42–43*).

Formula 3 parts St. John's Wort flowers and buds, 1 part Corn silk, 1 part Marshmallow root, 1 part Dandelion root, ½ part Vervain leaf.

Dosage Adults: 1 tsp (5ml) 3 times daily, plus a single night dose if woken. Children: over 2, adult dose; younger than 12, see page 45.

These herbs gently help maintain the bladder and kidneys, partly through their tannin (astringent) qualities and partly by relaxing the individual. The overall effect is soothing and cleansing, and relieves irritations in the bladder and kidneys.

RIGHT **Specially chosen herbs work together to create a soothing, healing formula.**

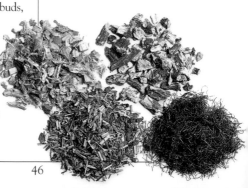

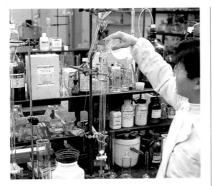

ABOVE *Scientists in laboratories are currently analysing herbs and their effects on the human body.*

RESEARCH RESULTS

In Germany more than 50% of cases of depression, anxiety, and sleep disorders are now treated with St. John's Wort; in sharp comparison, Prozac is used to treat just 2% of such cases in the country.

In August 1996, the *British Medical Journal* published the results of a trial by Klaus Linde and his associates of 23 controlled studies involving 1,757 depressed patients. In the analysis, researchers from both the US and Germany found that St. John's Wort worked nearly three times better than a placebo.

Currently St. John's Wort is undergoing trials in the US to explore whether it is effective as an antiviral agent.

CHRONIC VIRAL PROBLEMS

This formula made as a tincture is useful for easing deep, chronic, and long-term auto-immune problems.

Formula Equal parts of St. John's Wort buds and flowers, Marshmallow root, Siberian Ginseng root.

Dosage Adults: 1 tsp (5ml) 4 times daily. Children: over 12 years old, adult dose; younger than 12, see page 45.

St. John's Wort calms and balances an overactive and confused immune system.

Marshmallow root is a good tonic for the whole body and remedies the debilitating effects of viral problems.

Siberian Ginseng is good for treating chronic immune system problems. It will also help the other herbs and let the body's normal energy levels return slowly.

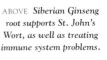

ABOVE *Siberian Ginseng root supports St. John's Wort, as well as treating immune system problems.*

MENOPAUSE

During the menopause a combination of symptoms are often present. A combined formula made as a tincture or into capsules is generally most effective, especially when the sufferer is experiencing depression, lethargy, and an overall lack of energy.

Formula 1 part each of St. John's Wort leaves and flowers, Black Cohosh root, Agnus Castus berries, and Sage, plus ½ part Passion flower.

Dosage 1 tsp (5ml) 3 or 4 times daily; night doses can also be taken if necessary.

St. John's Wort can ease menopausal depression, and Sage leaves will alleviate hot flushes.

The other herbs collectively balance the hormones and will ensure that the state of mind also regains balance.

This herbal formula should only be used with the support of a qualified herbalist.

NERVOUS DISORDERS

For nerve pains like shingles and Bell's palsy, for anxiety, insomnia, or tearfulness, for extreme tiredness and associated depression through sheer nervous exhaustion, this is an ideal formula made as a tincture or capsules. It nourishes the nervous system and uplifts the spirits.

Formula 2 parts St. John's Wort flowers and buds, 2 parts Oat straw, 2 parts Skullcap herb, 1 part Passion Flower, 1 part Pasque Flower, 1 part Vervain leaf, ¼ part Cayenne pods.

Dosage Adults: 1 tsp (5ml) 4 or 5 times daily. Not to be given to children unless supervised by a herbalist.

These herbs help to repair nerve endings and supply acetocyleine (a B vitamin important to nerve transmitter response). They relax, uplift, and feed the whole system.

LEFT **St. John's Wort formula raises the energy levels and combats nervous exhaustion.**

OVERALL DIGESTIVE TONIC

These herbs stimulate better working of the pancreas, liver, and stomach. They work best as a tincture because the taste in the mouth immediately activates the digestive juices. The herbs also contain bitters and stomach supportives.

Formula Equal parts of St. John's Wort buds and flowers, Gentian root, Chamomile flowers, Fennel seed, Echinacea root, Fenugreek seed, Meadowsweet herb.

Dosage Adults: 1 tsp (5ml) before meals, and again after meals if desired. Children: over 12 years old, adult dose; younger than 12, see page 45.

Meadowsweet balances the levels of acidity in the stomach.

SMOKING

This formula, made up either as a tincture or in capsules, can be effective for helping to give up smoking because it contains chemical components similar to those found in tobacco, in particular nicotine.

Formula 5 parts St. John's Wort buds and flowers, 1 part Lobelia herb.

Dosage Adults: ½–1 tsp (2.5–5ml) 3 times daily.

One of the reasons that nicotine is enjoyed by so many people is that it raises serotonin levels in the brain (see page 18). St. John's Wort's main chemical component (hypericin) maintains serotonin levels by preventing the premature depletion that some people experience.

Lobelia also has this effect, but is only available from a qualified herbal practitioner.

LEFT **A tonic based on St. John's Wort will help soothe away digestive problems.**

Conditions chart

THIS CHART is a guide to some of the ailments that St. John's Wort can treat, but it is not intended to replace other forms of treatment. Always consult your doctor or another qualified medical practitioner before embarking on a course of treatment.

NAME	INTERNAL USE	EXTERNAL USE
ANEMIA	Tincture, capsule	
ANXIETY	Tincture, capsule	
ARTHRITIS	Tincture, capsule	Cold-pressed oil, 3–4 times daily
AUTO-IMMUNE DISEASES	Tincture, capsule	
BED SORES		Cold-pressed oil, 3–4 times daily
BED-WETTING	Tincture, capsule	
BELL'S PALSY	Tincture, capsule	Cold-pressed oil
BLADDER DISORDERS	Tincture, capsule	
BLOOD CLEANSER	Tincture, capsule	
BRONCHITIS	Tincture, capsule	
BRUISES		Cold-pressed oil, 5–6 times daily
BURNS	Tincture, capsule	Cold-pressed oil, 3–4 times daily
BURSITIS	Tincture, capsule	Cold-pressed oil, 3–4 times daily

NAME	INTERNAL USE	EXTERNAL USE
CANDIDA	Tincture (boil off the alcohol with hot water), capsule	Cold-pressed oil (you can insert the oil on a tampon for 1 hour) once daily
CHEST CONGESTION	Tincture, capsule	Cold-pressed oil, 3 times daily
COMMON COLD	Tincture, capsule	
COLD SORES	Tincture, capsule	Cold-pressed oil, poultice (can mix with other herbs) at night
DEPRESSION	Tincture, capsule	
DERMATITIS		Cold-pressed oil or ointment, as and when needed
DIARRHEA	Tincture, capsule	
DIGESTIVE AID	Tincture, capsule	
FROZEN SHOULDER		Cold-pressed oil or ointment, as and when needed
GASTROENTERITIS	Tincture, capsule	
GLANDULAR FEVER	Tincture, capsule	
HEADACHES – TENSION	Tincture, capsule	Cold-pressed oil on temples, hourly
HERPES	Tincture, capsule	Cold-pressed oil or ointment, hourly
IMPETIGO		Cold-pressed oil, 4–5 times daily

NAME	INTERNAL USE	EXTERNAL USE
INCONTINENCE	Tincture, capsule	
INDIGESTION	Tincture, capsule	
INFLAMMATION Useful for acute trauma but also where aberrations of natural immune system response have been produced for example in allergies and some chronic diseases	Tincture, capsule	Cold-pressed oil or ointment, as and when needed
INFLUENZA	Tincture, capsule	
INSOMNIA	Tincture, capsule, at night	
JAUNDICE	Tincture, capsule	
MASTITIS	Tincture, capsule	Cold-pressed oil, 2–3 times daily
MENOPAUSE Menopausal headaches and associated depression	Tincture, capsule	
NEURALGIA	Tincture, capsule	Cold-pressed oil, as and when needed
PEPTIC ULCER	Cold-pressed oil	
PREMENSTRUAL TENSION/SYNDROME	Tincture, capsule	
PSORIASIS		Cold-pressed oil, 3–4 times daily
SCIATICA		Cold-pressed oil, 3-4 times daily
SHAKING PALSY	Tincture, capsule	Cold-pressed oil, twice daily

NAME	INTERNAL USE	EXTERNAL USE
SHINGLES	Tincture, capsule	Cold-pressed oil, twice daily
SINUSITIS	Tincture, capsule	
SLEEP DISORDERS	Tincture, capsule	
SPONDYLITIS		Massage spine with cold-pressed oil, 4–5 times daily
STOMATITIS	Gargle tincture before swallowing	
SUNBURN		Cold-pressed oil, hourly
TOOTH PAIN	Gargle tincture before swallowing	Dab cold-pressed oil on abscess with cotton wool
ULCERS (EXTERNAL)		cold-pressed oil x 2 daily
ULCERS (INTERNAL)	Tincture, capsule	
URTICARIA		Cold-pressed oil, 5–6 times daily
UTERINE CRAMPING	Tincture, capsule	
VAGINITIS		Cold-pressed oil (insert the oil on a tampon for 1 hour)
WORMS	Tincture, capsule	

How St. John's Wort works

ST. JOHN'S WORT *has many naturally occurring components, most notably naphthodianthrones and their derivatives hypericin and pseudohypericin. It also contains flavonoids, tannins, and phytosterols, plus various amino acids and essential oils.*

While climate, soil, species, and other factors will determine the amounts in which St. John's Wort's many compounds are found, researchers and herbalists largely agree that the effects of the herb are due to an interaction between all of its chemical constituents – and not just one or two key components.

MAIN EFFECTS

🌺 By inhibiting the immune system response of producing lymphocytes and T-cells, St. John's Wort's chemistry produces an anti-inflammatory effect. This can be helpful where the immune system's response has become excessive or out of control, as in the case of some chronic diseases.

🌺 All the compounds contained in St. John's Wort seem to increase deep sleep but slightly decrease REM (rapid eye movement) sleep. Deep sleep provides our nighttime rest, while in REM sleep we dream.

🌺 The compounds in St. John's Wort also work against viruses by attacking the cellular membrane and inhibiting the receptor activity that are involved in abnormal growth (helpful for antiviral and antibacterial activities).

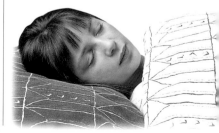

BELOW *St. John's Wort seems to lengthen spells of deep sleep.*

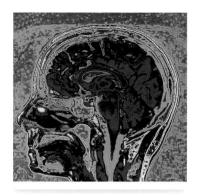

ABOVE *Scans have been carried out into the effects of St. John's Wort on the sleeping brain.*

❋ The flavonoids are believed to aid the sedative effects of the herb, while others help produce some of its antidepressant effects.

❋ The tannins may well help St. John's Wort to be effective for burns and rapid healing by providing extra oxygen. They may also support its anti-inflammatory quality.

❋ Phytosterols are plant steroids that can be translated into human steroids by bacteria in the gut. They can be used for pain relief and as an anti-inflammatory where "human" steroids are missing, such as in the adrenal glands.

❋ The herb's amino acids are the building blocks for neurotransmitters. They help to produce better connections, and subsequently calm and balance the activity of the brain.

❋ St. John's Wort essential oils contribute vital healing and sedative qualities.

CASE STUDY: PAIN RELIEF

David's left shoulder had been stiff and sore for some time. To make matters worse, he had to drive for up to three hours a day, and the pain in his shoulder made it very difficult for him to drive his car. The ibuprofen (muscular relaxant drug) he was taking didn't help despite the fact that it was the maximum dose permissible. His daughter suggested rubbing St. John's Wort into the shoulder twice daily.

After four days of using the red oil he felt some real changes and a week later he was able to tell his daughter that it was making a significant difference and that he would willingly continue to use it. He also decided to phase out the use of his pain management pills.

Glossary

AERIAL PARTS

Parts of a plant that grow above the ground.

ANTISPASMODIC

Herb that limits, corrects, and prevents excessive involuntary muscular contractions.

ANTIOXIDANTS

Substances found particularly in high-chlorophyll foods that protect the cells from the free radicals (damaging atoms) and reduce the risk of some serious diseases.

BELL'S PALSY

Paralysis of the facial nerve.

BURSITIS

Inflammation of the bursae, small sacs of fibrous tissue that reduce friction over ligaments and tendons.

DECOCTION

Method of preparing and preserving herbs in water.

DOPAMINERGIC ACTIVITY

Action of the hormone dopamine that prevents the hormone prolactin from secreting milk by the mammary glands.

ESTROGEN

Female reproductive hormone, the production of which decreases during the menopause.

FIBROSITIS

Inflammation of fibrous connective tissue that causes muscular pain and stiffness.

FLAVONOIDS

Compounds in plants that are responsible for a wide range of actions that include reducing inflammation and fighting fungus.

FREE RADICALS

Highly reactive particles that damage cell membranes, DNA, and other cell structures.

HYPOGLYCEMIC

Person suffering from hypoglycemia (low blood sugar).

HYPOTHALAMUS

Thermoregulatory mechanism of the brain that also controls the pituitary gland.

IMMUNITY

Capacity and function of the body to fend off foreign bodies, and/or to disarm and eject them.

IMPETIGO
Bacterial infection of the outer layers of the skin.

INFUSION
Method of releasing a herb's flavor and chemicals through immersion in boiling water.

LYMPHOCYTE
Type of white blood cell.

MASTITIS
Inflammation of the breast.

NEURALGIA
Intense pain that originates in any nerve.

NEUROTRANSMITTERS
Molecules released into the synaptic cleft in response to a nerve impulse.

PROGESTERONE
Female hormone of the second stage of the menstrual cycle that prepares for and supports pregnancy.

PSORIASIS
A chronic skin disease in which scaly pink patches form on the scalp, knees, elbows, and other parts of the body.

SCIATICA
Pain felt down the back, and outer side of the thigh, leg, and foot. It is usually caused by degeneration of an intervertebral disc.

SHAKING PALSY
Disturbance of voluntary movement affecting mobility, and speech.

SPONDYLITIS
Degenerative process of the vertebrae and joints between them.

STOMATITIS
Inflammation of the mucus membrane of the mouth.

T-CELLS
Immune system cells that play several roles in the body's defences.

TINCTURE
Plant medicine prepared by soaking herbs in alcohol and water.

TOPICAL
Application of herbs to the surface of the body as opposed to being taken internally.

URTICARIA (NETTLE RASH, HIVES)
Manifestation of an allergic reaction.

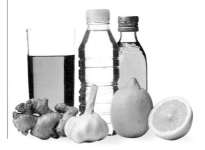

Further reading

BRITISH HERBAL PHARMACOPOEIA 1983 AND 1996 (British Herbal Medical Association, 1996)

THE COMPLETE ILLUSTRATED HOLISTIC HERBAL, *David Hoffmann* (Element Books Limited, 1996)

CURES FROM THE LAST CHANCE CLINIC, *Richard Schulze* (University of Natural Healing, Virginia, 1995)

ENCYCLOPAEDIA OF HERBS AND HERBALISM, *Malcolm Stuart* (Black Cat, 1987)

ENCYCLOPAEDIA OF HERBS AND THEIR USES, *Deni Bown* (Dorling Kindersley, 1995)

ENCYCLOPAEDIA OF MEDICINAL PLANTS, *Andrew Chevallier* (Dorling Kindersley, 1996)

ESSENTIAL SCIENCE CHEMISTRY, *Freemantle & Tidy* (Oxford University Press, 1993)

GARDENER'S DICTIONARY OF PLANT NAMES, *Dr. William T. Stearn* (Cassell, 1983)

HERBAL MEDICINE MAKER'S HANDBOOK, *James Green* (Wildlife & Green Publications, 1990)

HERBAL PHARMACOLOGY, *Christopher Hobbs* (Botanica Press, 1990)

HERBAL RENAISSANCE, *Steven Foster* (Healing Arts Press, 1984)

HYPERICUM PERFORATUM (review published by American Botanical Council & Herb Research Foundation, Herbalgram No 18/19, Fall 1998 and Winter 1989)

MANUAL OF CONVENTIONAL MEDICINE FOR ALTERNATIVE PRACTITIONERS, *Stephen Gascoigne* (Jigame Press, 1994)

NATURAL PROZAC PROGRAM, *Jonathan Zuess MD* (Three Rivers Press, 1997)

NUTRITIONAL HERBOLOGY *Mark Pederson* (Wendell W. Whitman Company, 1994)

OUT OF THIS EARTH, *Simon Mills* (Viking, 991)

ST. JOHN'S WORT (Hypericum perforatum and Hypericum angustifolia), *Camilla Cracchiolo* (RN, 1997)

SCHOOL OF NATURAL HEALING, *Dr. Christopher* (Christopher Publications, 1976)

SPIRITUAL PROPERTIES OF HERBS, *Gurudas* (Cassandra Press, 1988)

TEXTBOOK OF ADVANCED HERBOLOGY, *Terry Willard* (Wild Rose College of Natural Healing, 1992)

TEXTBOOK OF MODERN HERBOLOGY, *Terry Willard* (Wild Rose College of Natural Healing, Alberta, 1993)

WILD FLOWERS OF BRITAIN AND NORTHERN EUROPE, *Alistair & Richard Fitter & Marjorie Blamey* (Collins, 1985)

Useful addresses

ASSOCIATIONS AND SOCIETIES

**British Herbal Medicine
Association (B.H.M.A)**
Sun House, Church Street, Stroud,
Glos. GL5 1JL, UK
Tel: 011 44 1453–751389
Fax: 011 44 1453–751402
Works with the Medicine Control
Agency to promote high standards of
quality and safety of herbal medicine

Herb Society
Deddington Hill Farm,
Warmington, Banbury,
Oxon OX17 1XB, UK
Tel: 011 44 1295–692000
Fax: 011 44 1295–692004
Educational charity that disseminates
information about herbs and
organizes workshops

**The Wild Plant Conservation
Charity**
The Natural History Museum,
Cromwell Road,
London SW7 5BD, UK
Tel: 011 44 171–938 9123
Registered charity to save British
wild plants

SUPPLIERS IN THE UK

Baldwin & Company
171–173 Walworth Road,
London SE17 1RW, UK
Tel: 011 44 171–703 5550
Herbs, storage bottles, jars, and
containers available

Hambleden Herbs
Court Farm, Milverton,
Somerset TA4 1NF, UK
Tel: 011 44 1823–401205
Organic herbs by mail order

Herbs, Hands, Healing
The Cabins, Station Warehouse,
Station Road, Pulham Market,
Norfolk IP21 4XF, UK
Tel: 011 44 1379–608007
Tel/fax: 011 44 1379–608201
Herbal formulas, organic herbs,
and Superfood

SUPPLIERS/SCHOOLS IN THE USA

American Botanical Pharmacy
PO Box 3027, Santa Monica,
CA 90408, USA
Tel/fax: 1310 453–1987
Manufacturer and distributor of
herbal products; runs training courses

Blessed Herbs
109 Barre Plains Road,
Oakham,
MA 01068, USA
Tel: 1800 489–4372
Dried bulk herbs are available by
mail order in order to make your
own preparations

United Plant Savers
PO Box 420,
E. Barre,
VT 05649, USA
Aims to preserve wild Native
American medicinal plants

Other Healing Herb Books
in the Nutshell Series

❧

ECHINACEA
ECHINACEA ANGUSTIFOLIA
ECHINACEA PURPUREA

❧

GARLIC
ALLIUM SATIVUM

❧

GINKGO
GINKGO BILOBA

❧

GINSENG
ELEUTHEROCOCCUS SENTICOSUS

❧

HAWTHORN
CRATAEGUS MONOGYNA

❧

MARIGOLD
CALENDULA OFFICINALIS

❧

SAW PALMETTO
SERENOA SERRULATA

❧